courageous

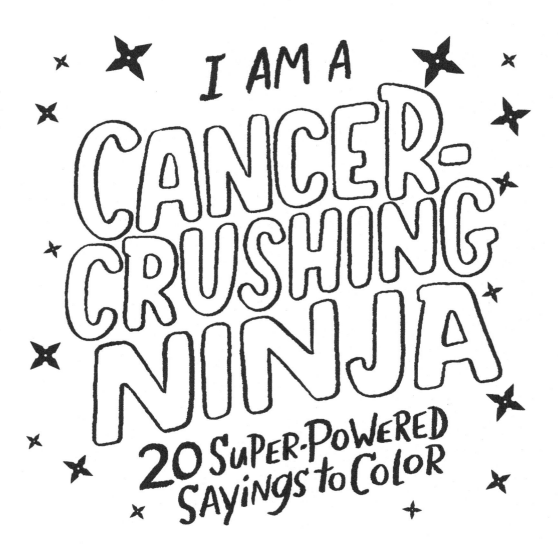

I AM A
CANCER-
CRUSHING
NINJA
20 Super-Powered
Sayings to Color

kathyWELLER

I Am A Cancer-Crushing Ninja: 20 Super-Powered Sayings To Color ©2018 Kathy Weller

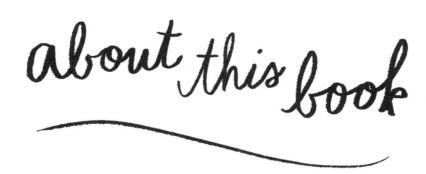

about this book

My first cancer coloring book, I Am A Cancer Warrior, was inspired by a close member of my family who had cancer. Even though I couldn't physically be there, I got creative with other ways I could help support him through his treatment. I share that story in the beginning of that book.

This, my second cancer coloring book, was inspired by YOU. Many of you have been using I Am A Cancer Warrior throughout your own diagnosis and treatment. You all have blown me away with your motivation, inspiration and positivity! You've shared positive feedback, enthusiasm, and appreciation for I Am A Cancer Warrior on social media. You've reached out to me personally, to let me know what it's meant to you. You have inspired me EVERY day and in EVERY way, since I first put I Am A Cancer Warrior out there for you to discover and enjoy. THANK YOU.

For a long time, I've wanted to do a follow-up coloring book for you. I wanted it to be "EXTRA"— in both the art AND in the motivational sayings! Hey, I personally think I've succeeded with this one... but YOU are the true judge of that! So please, don't be shy to let me know what you think!

Anyway, I'm SO thrilled that I Am A Cancer-Crushing Ninja is in your hands right now! More strong, motivational and meaningful sayings, more fun art to color, more SUPPORT for YOU to kick cancer butt!

I hope this book makes you smile inside-out and FEEL THE POWER! I know it's incredibly hard. That's why this book is here for ya. PLEASE keep the fire of your fight stoked. I'm WITH YOU to BEAT that stupid cancer and leave it in the DUST! Stay strong. Stay focused. And, keep coloring. Hugs to you!

XO,
Kathy

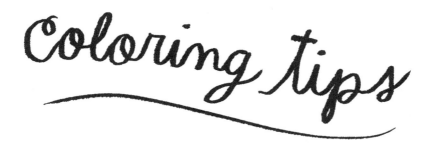

Coloring tips

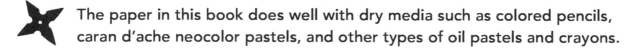
The paper in this book does well with dry media such as colored pencils, caran d'ache neocolor pastels, and other types of oil pastels and crayons.

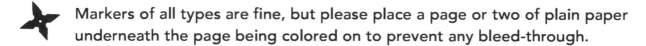
Markers of all types are fine, but please place a page or two of plain paper underneath the page being colored on to prevent any bleed-through.

The images to color are printed on one side of the paper, with the other side left intentionally blank.

Some of the illustrations feature darker, thicker black lines. They're there for variety, to emphasize parts of the design, and to give you flexibility for exploration with opaque drawing media, like gel pens and crayons!

I made an effort to balance each coloring design with a little extra space in the book binding area. This was done to make it easier for you to cut the page out, if you wish to.

Have fun!

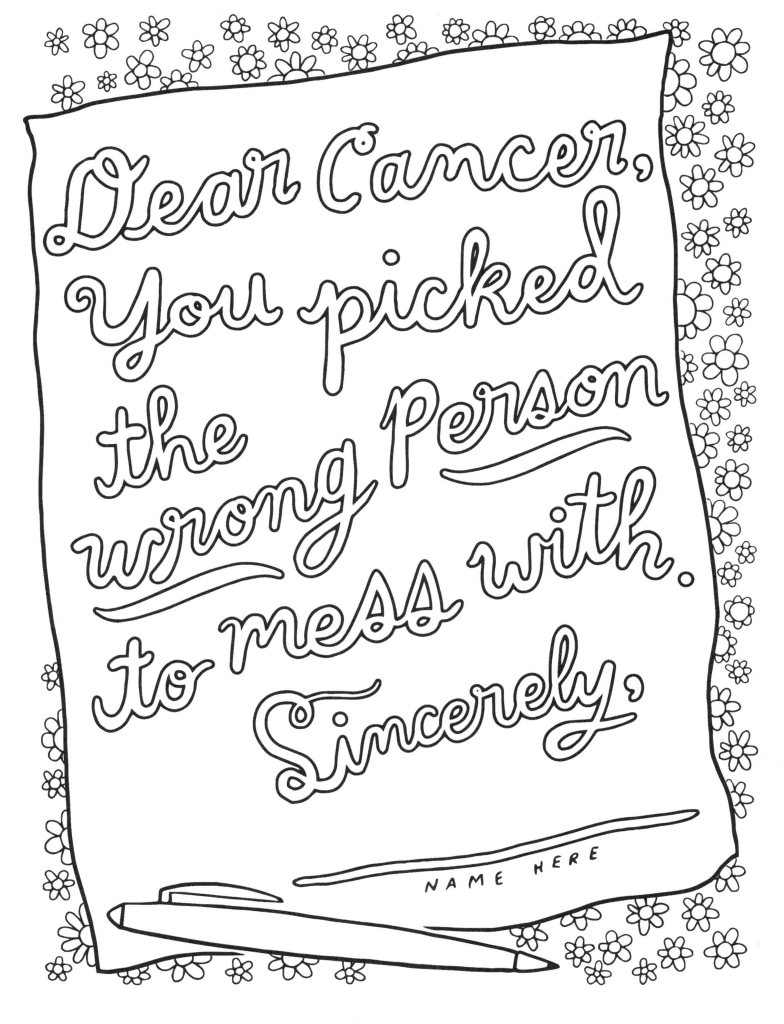

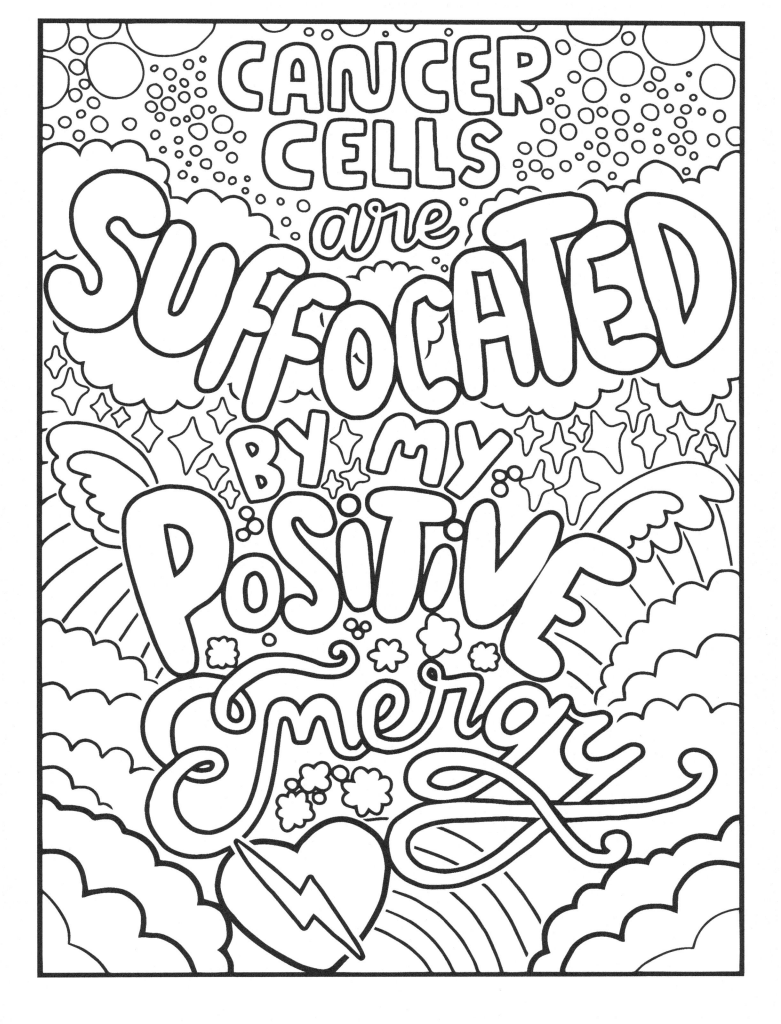

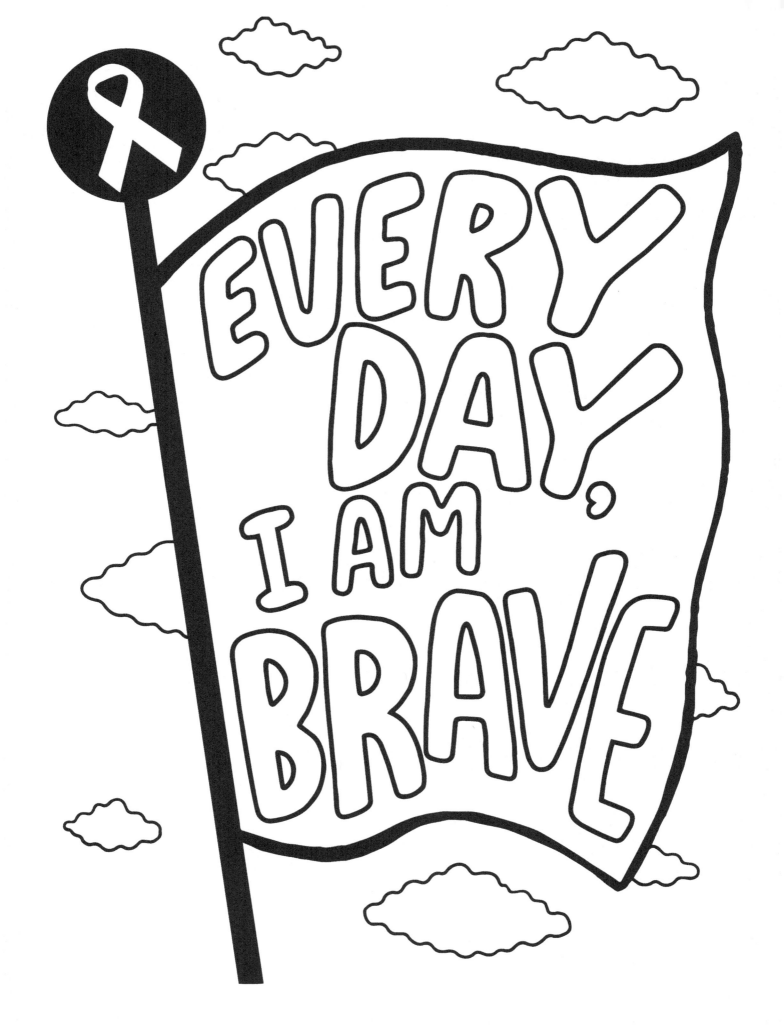

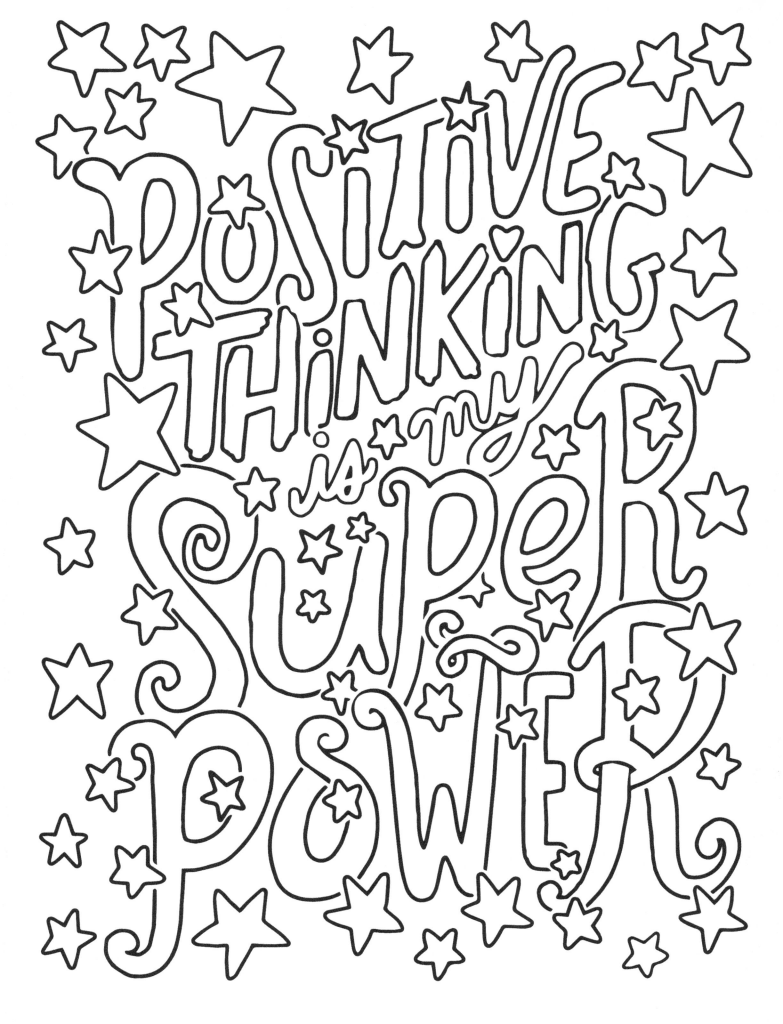

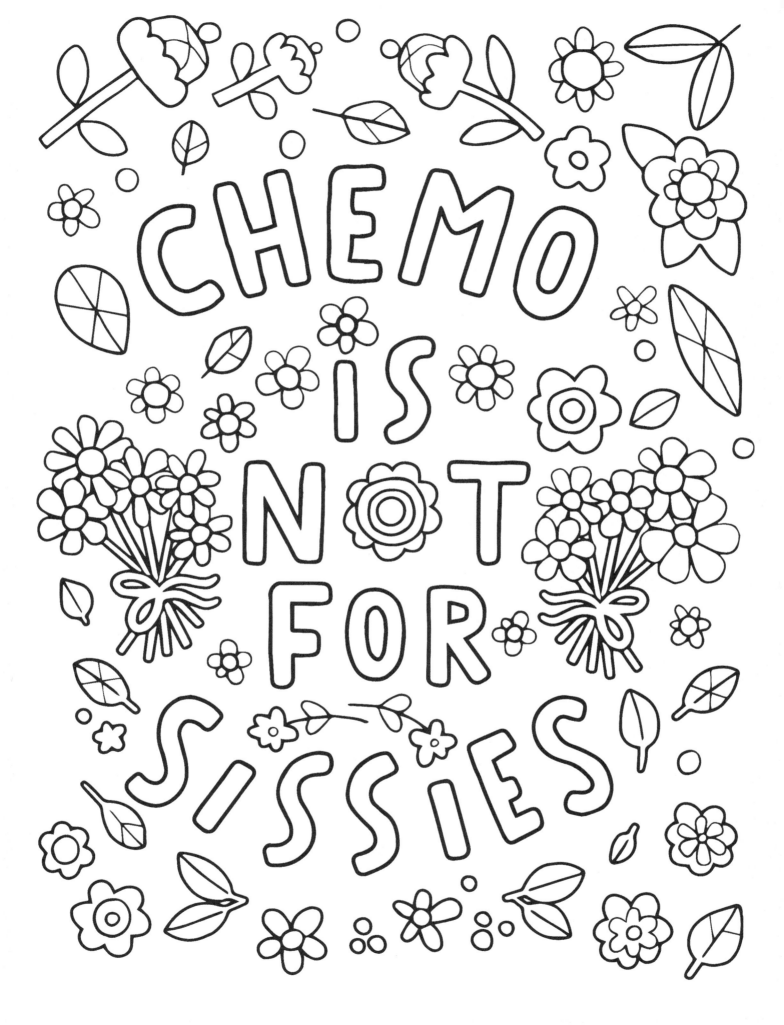

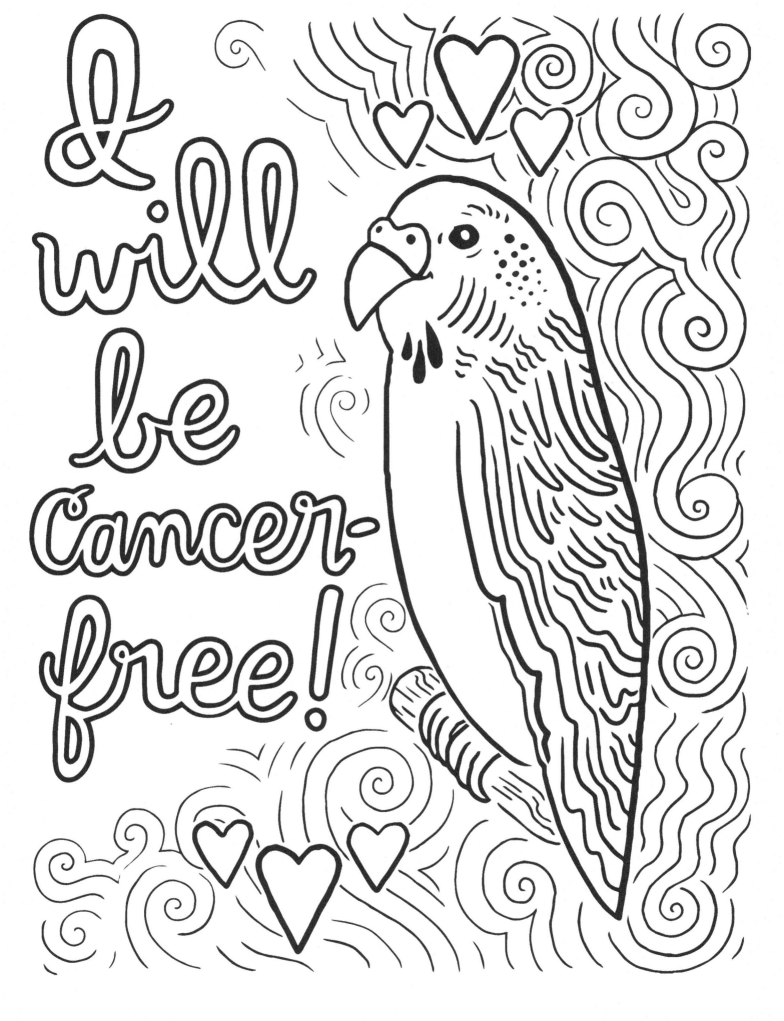

I will be cancer-free!

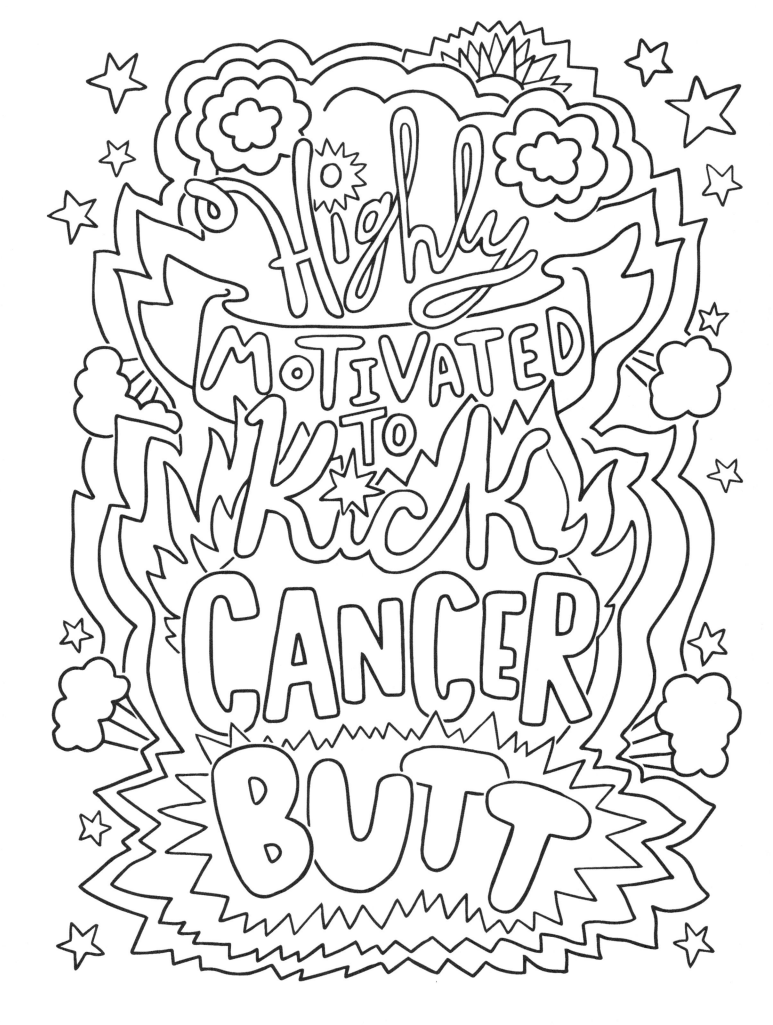

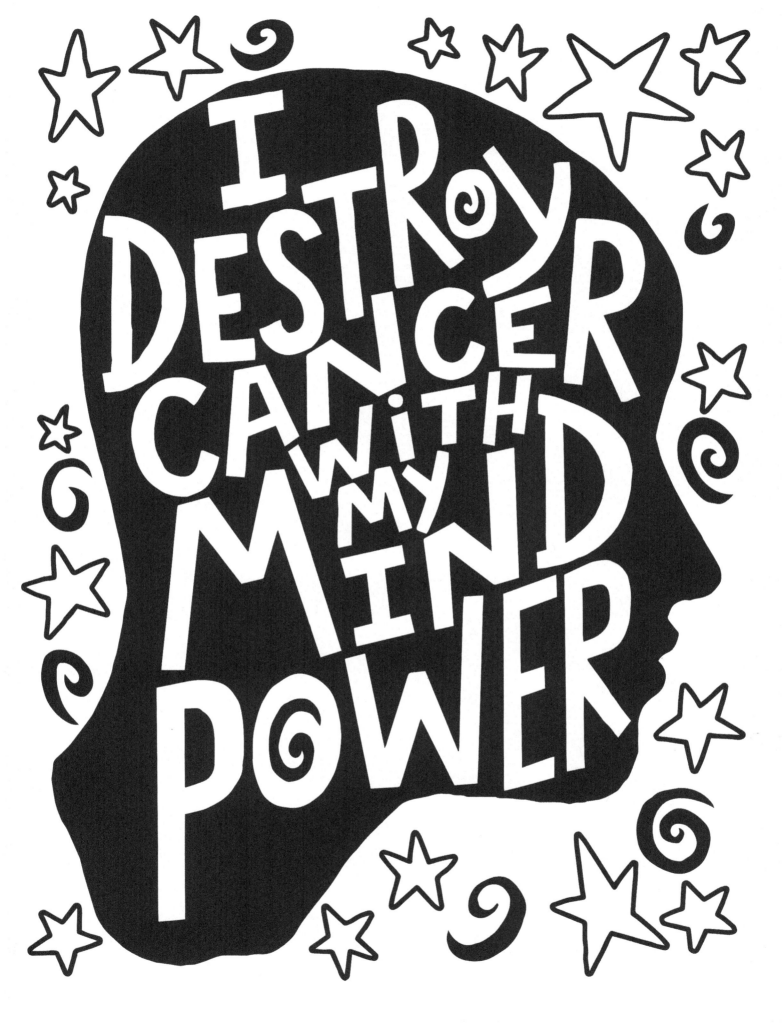

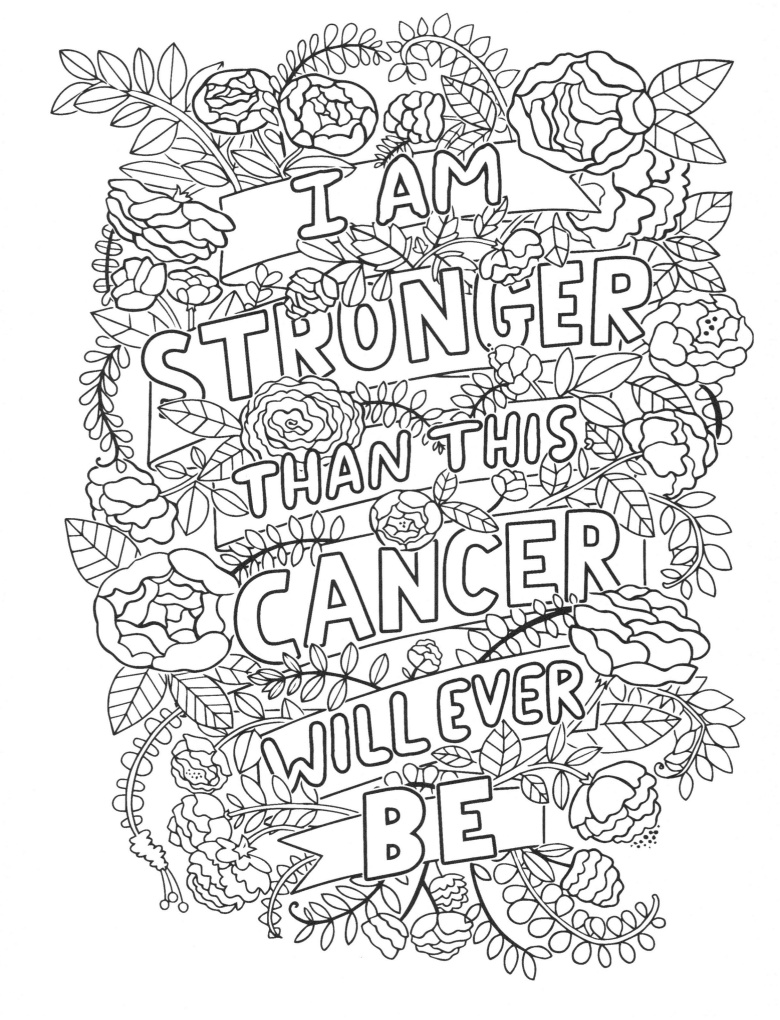

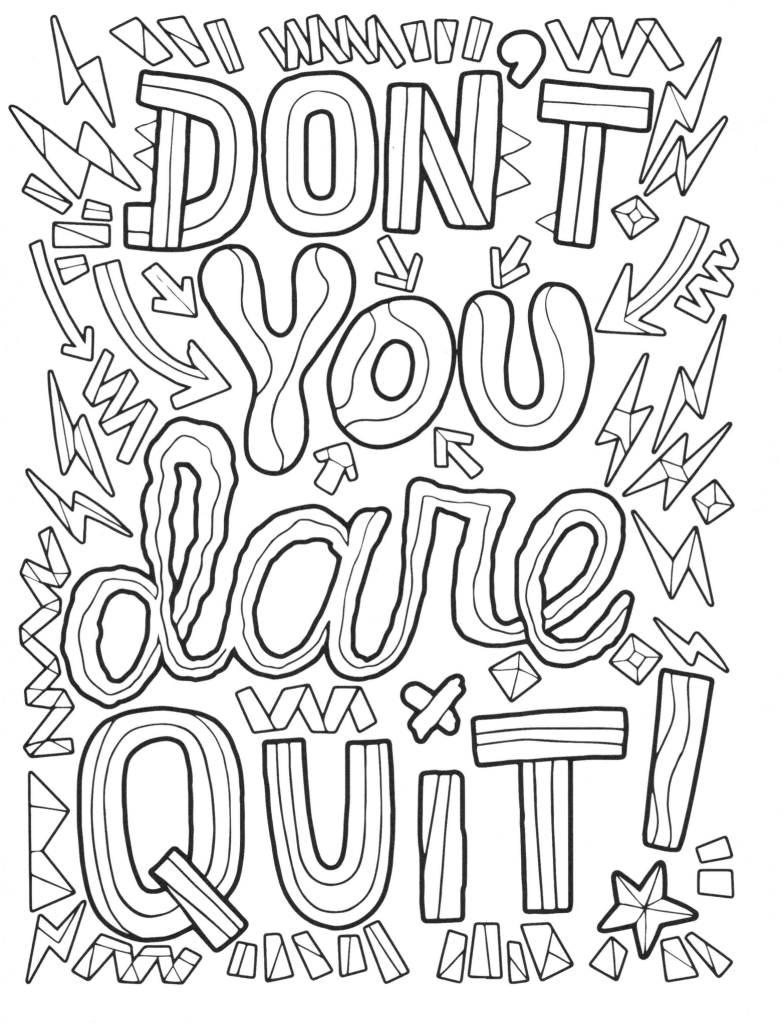

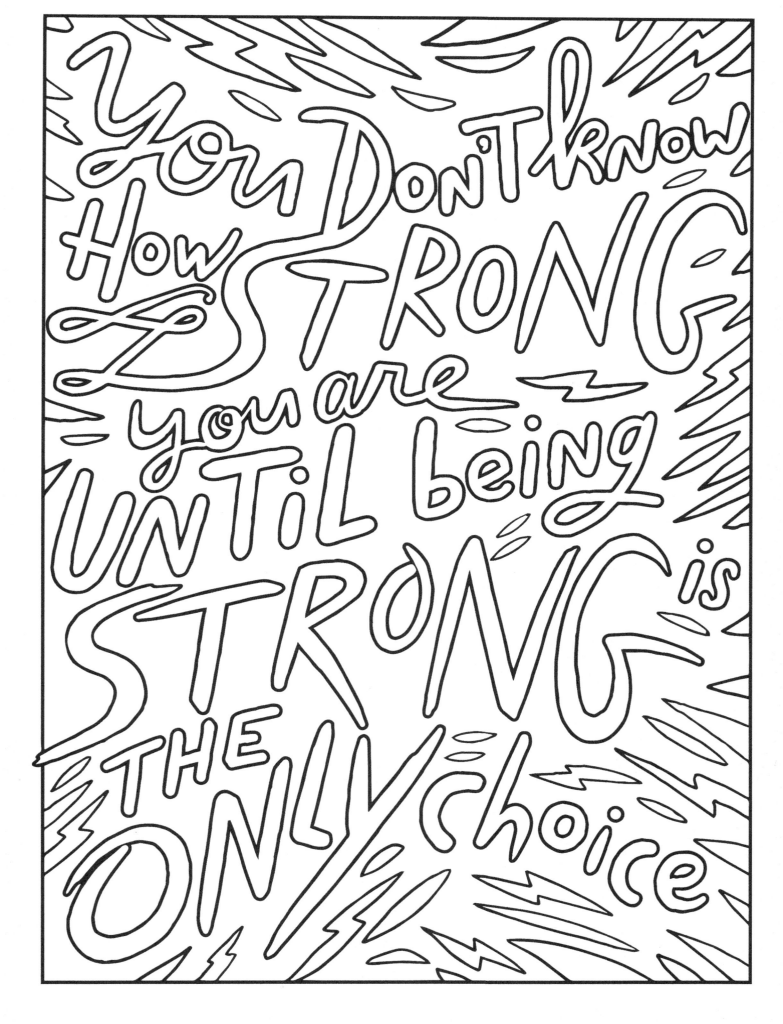

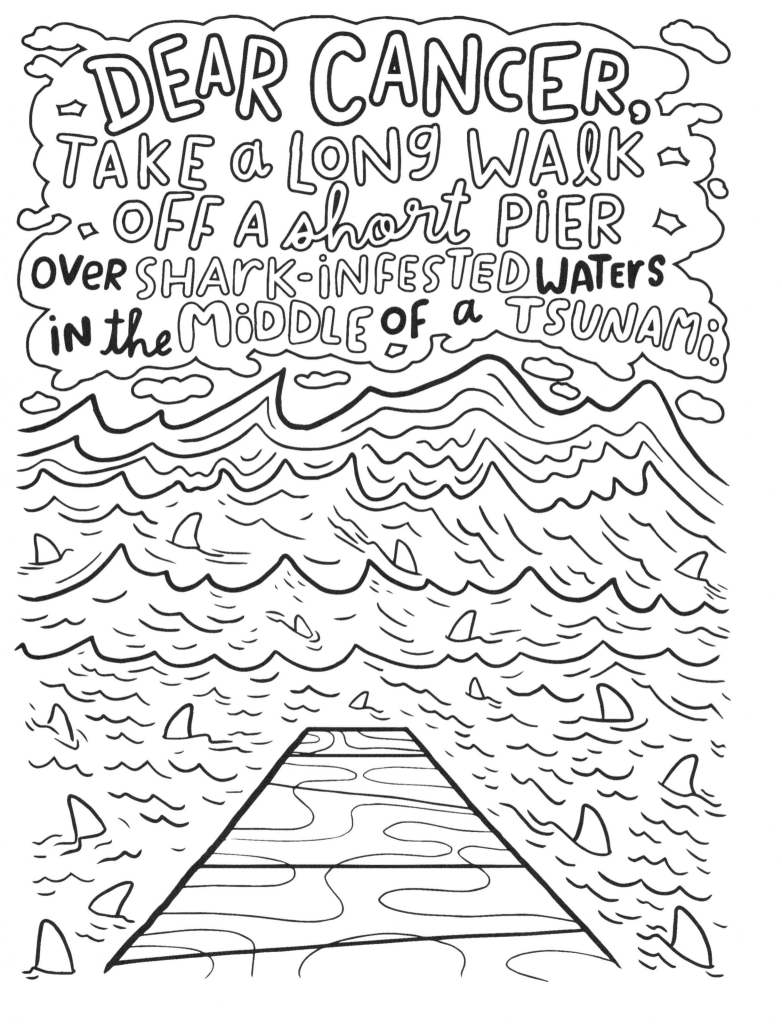

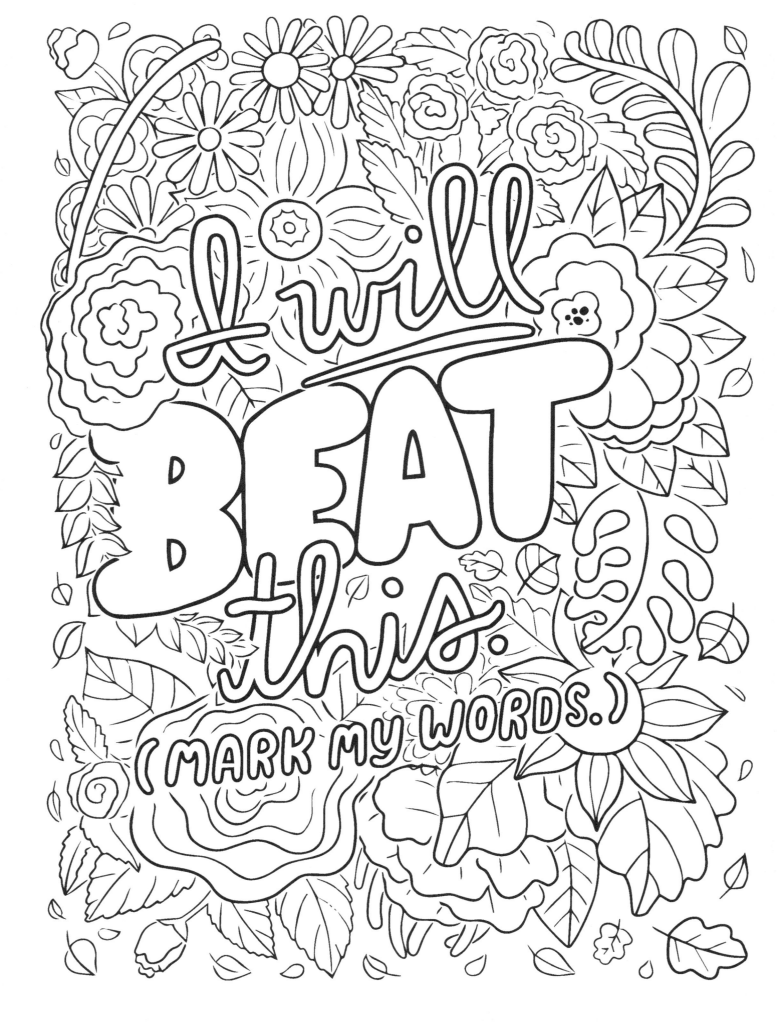

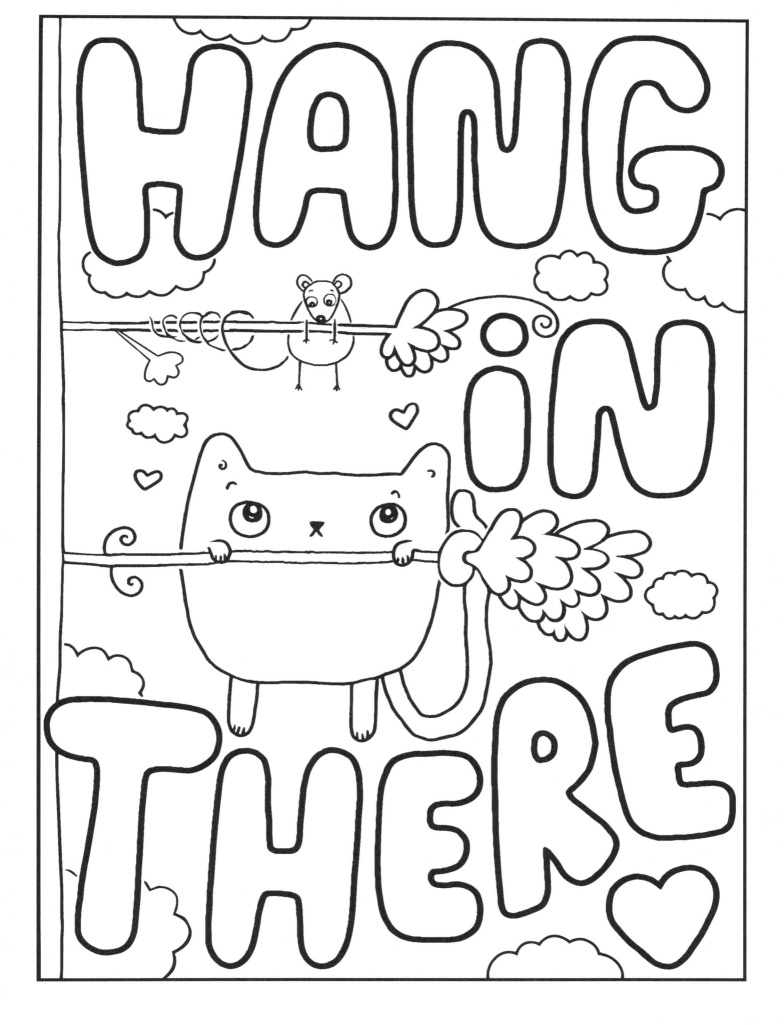

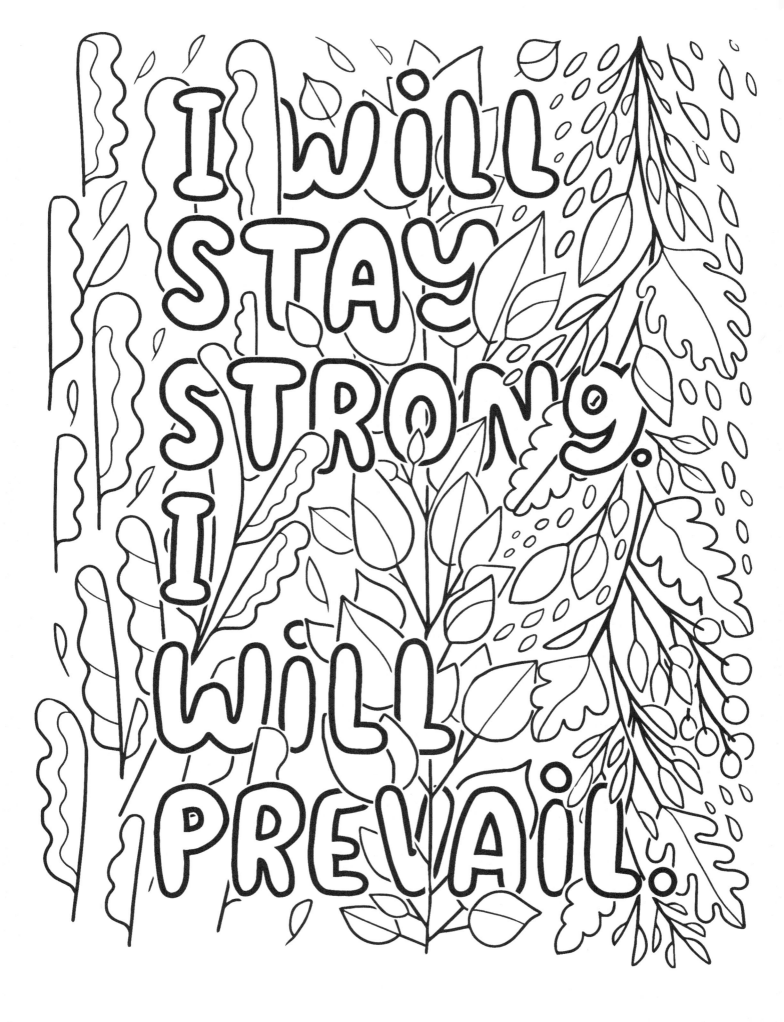

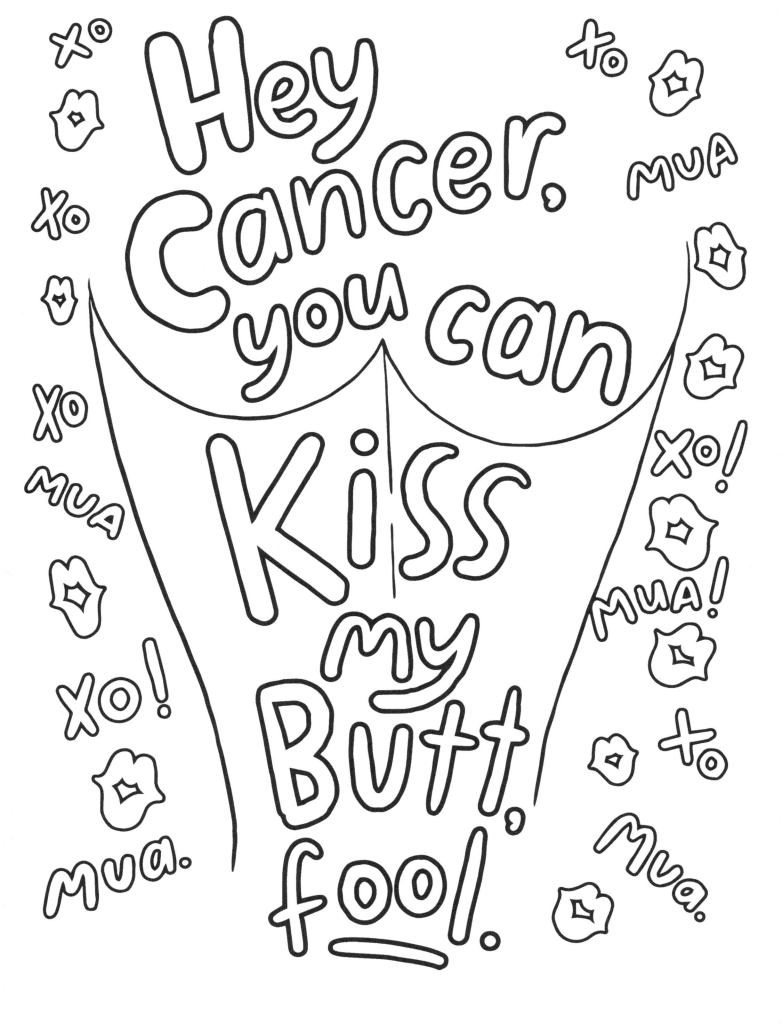

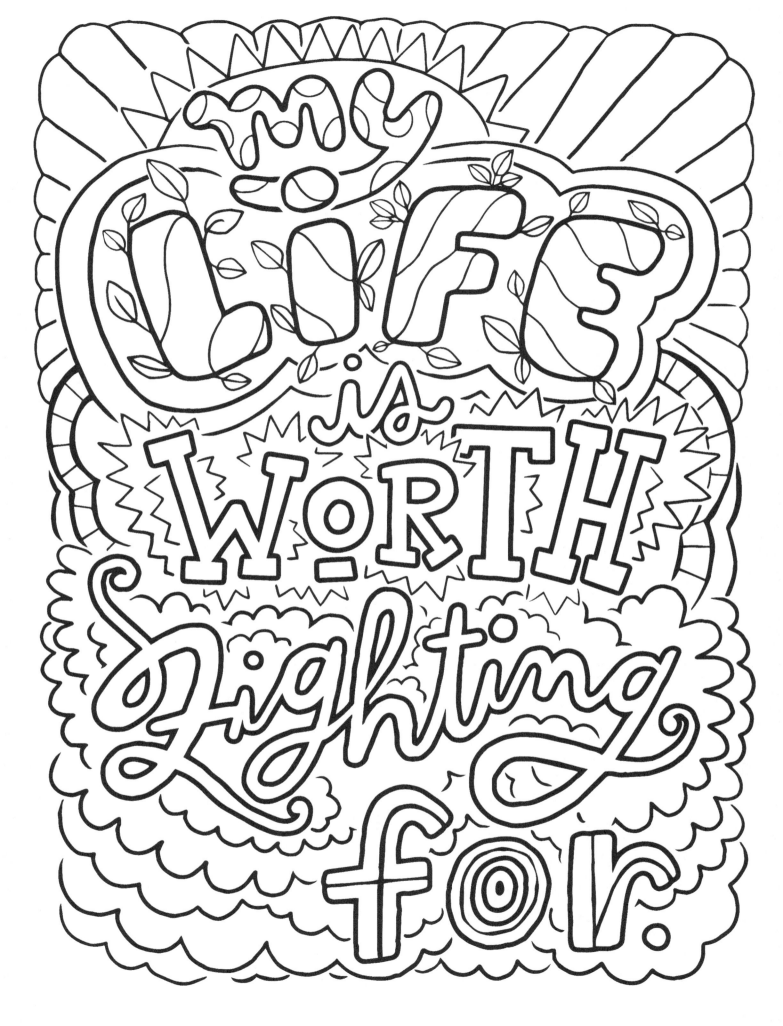

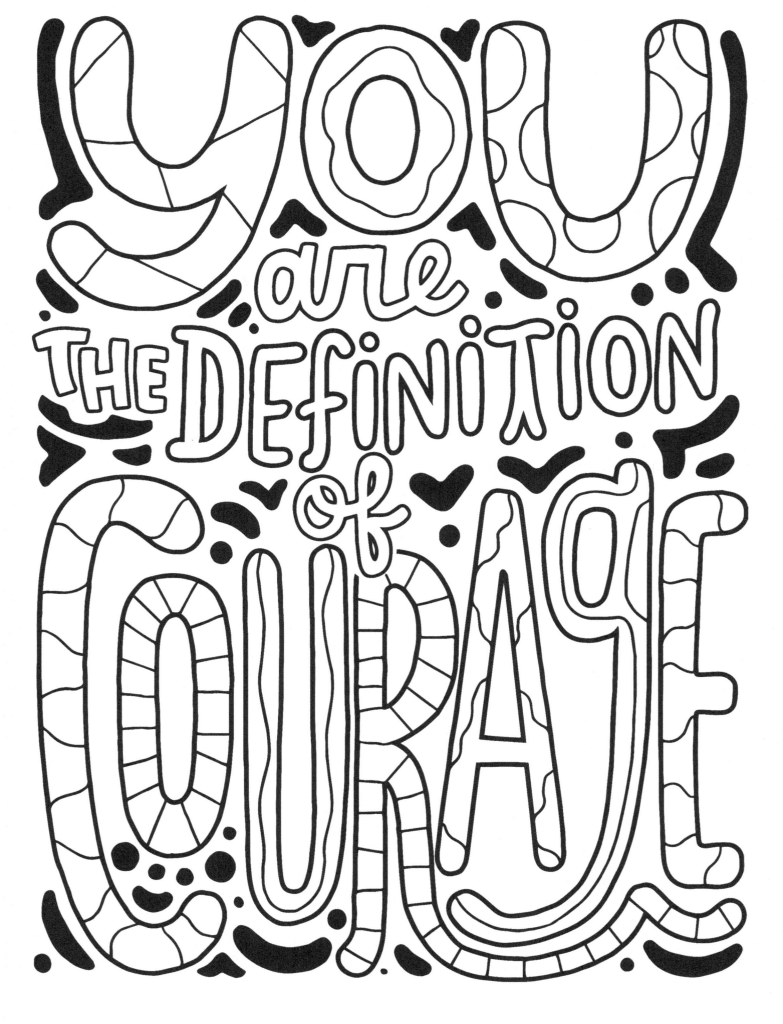

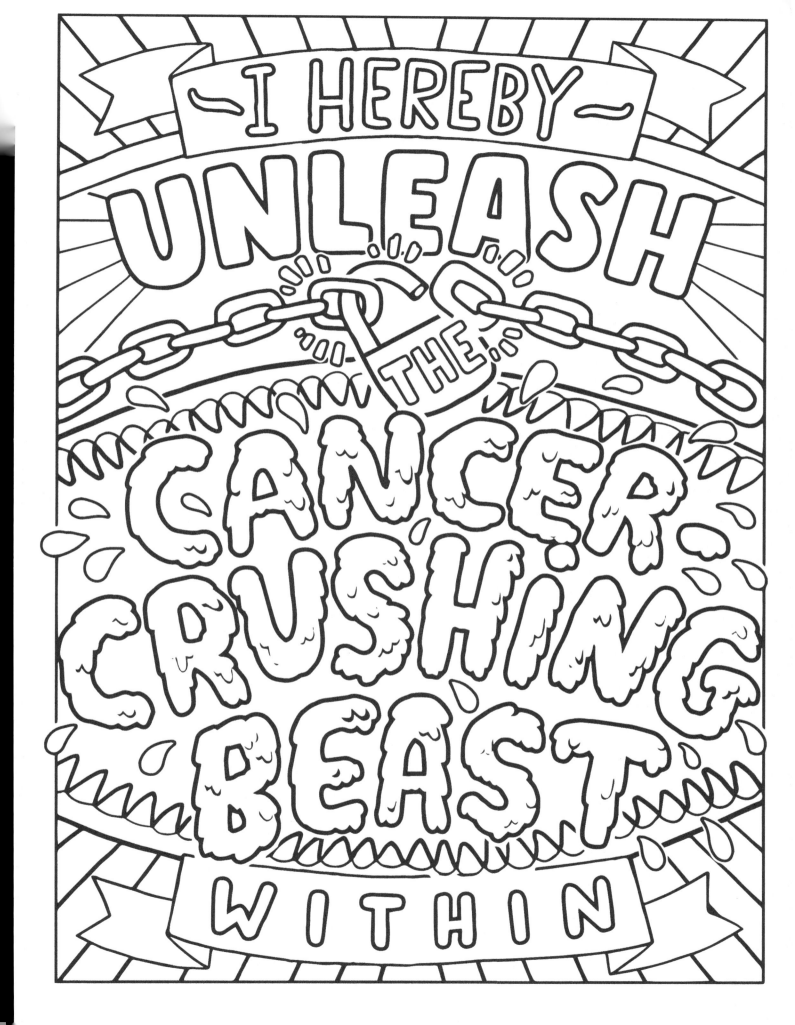

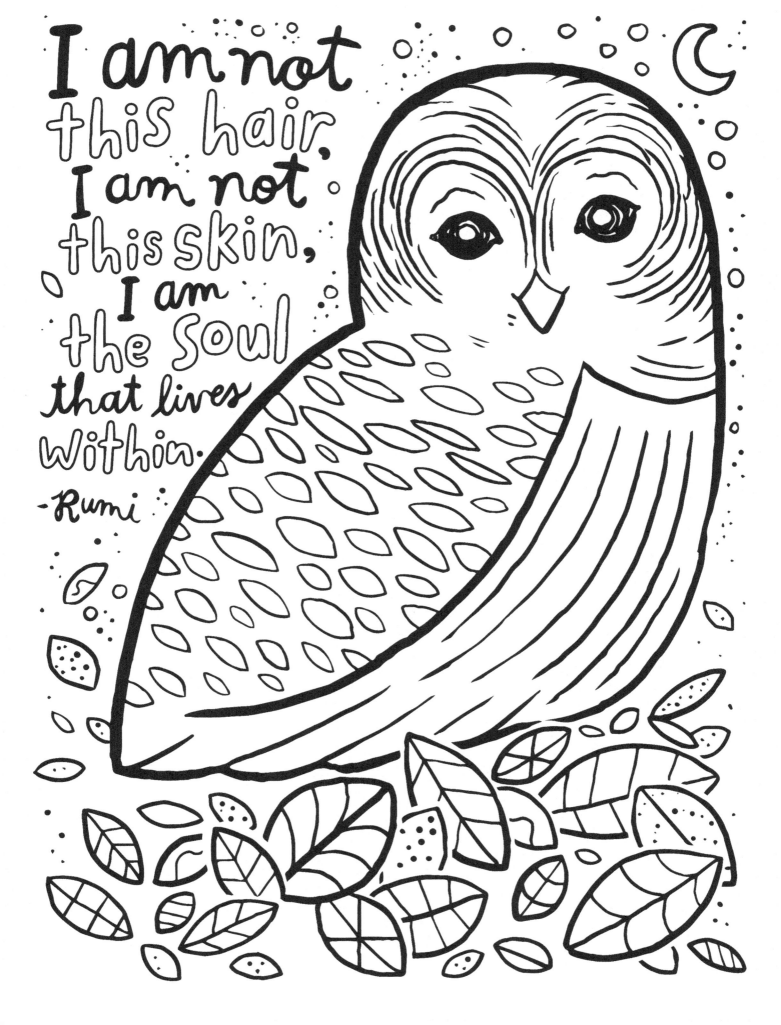

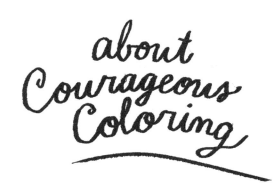

about Courageous Coloring

I started Couageous Coloring to encourage creative exploration and discovery for everyone, without self-criticism or judgement.
Get encouraged, motivated, and inspired with Courageous Coloring!

 I Am A Cancer-Crushing Ninja is the fourth coloring book in this series.

Also available:

 I Am A Cancer Warrior

 I Am A Chronic Illness Crusader

 I Am A Kidney Disease Warrior

For more releases, please visit

CourageousColoring.com

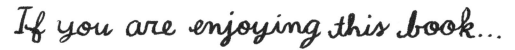

If you are enjoying this book...

Please leave an Amazon review. People just like you are shopping Amazon right now, looking for a coloring book just like this one. The more reviews this book has, the more visible Amazon will make it to others shopping for similar books. Reviews that include photos or videos of your beautiful coloring pages are extremely appreciated!!

let's connect!

Coloring books
courageouscoloring.com
shop.kathyweller.com
kathywellerart.etsy.com

facebook
facebook.com/**kathywellerart**

Twitter
twitter.com/**kathywellerart**
twitter.com/**courageouscolor**

Instagram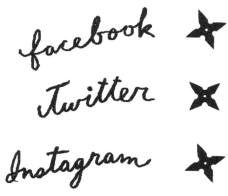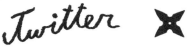
instagram.com/**kathywellerart**
instagram.com/**courageouscoloring**
instagram.com/**shopkathyweller**

main site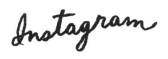
kathyweller.com

art videos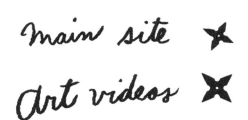
youtube.com/**kathywellerart**

Made in the USA
Monee, IL
27 January 2020